WOMAN MEDICINE
Vitex Agnus-Castus

by Simon Mills
MA FNIMH

Published by
Amberwood Publishing Ltd
Guildford, England

PLANTLIFE

The Natural History Museum, Cromwell Road, London SW7 5BD

Registered Charity No. 328576

Amberwood Publishing supports the Plantlife Charity,
Britain's only charity exclusively dedicated to saving wild plants.

ISBN 0-9517723-3-3

Cover production by Howland Northover

Printed in Great Britain

CONTENTS

Page No

1. WOMAN MEDICINE 9

2. THE OVARIAN CLOCK AND HORMONAL BALANCE 15

3. AGNUS-CASTUS IN MODERN MEDICINE ... 25

4. AGNUS-CASTUS: THE CLINICAL POTENTIAL ... 33

5. SOURCE AND DOSAGE 43

6. INDEX 45

Note to Reader

About the Author

Simon Mills was born in France and attended schools in London, Jordan and New Zealand before reading medical sciences at Cambridge University. After graduation he moved to study the practice of medical herbalism with the National Institute of Medical Herbalists, founded in 1864 and the oldest professional body of medical herbalists in the western world. He graduated from its 4-year training course and set up in practice in 1977.

He has since been Director of Research for the Institute and for six years their President. He played an active part in setting new professional standards for the wide spectrum of complementary medicine and was the first Chairman of the Council for Complementary and Alternative Medicine (CCAM), the first national association of major professional bodies in the field, and was a founder trustee of the first research organisation, the Research Council for Complementary Medicine (RCCM).

Since 1983 he has been a Council member of the British Herbal Medicine Association (BHMA), the body primarily engaged in setting public standards for herbal medicines, and negotiating with Government on such matters. In this role he was on the revision committee for the British Herbal Pharmacopoeia, which set unprecedented standards for medicinal plants and is used by government departments around the world. He is also a BHMA delegate to the European Scientific Cooperative on Phytotherapy (ESCOP) a European association of national organisations concerned with promoting at EC level, harmonised standards for the quality, safety and efficacy of medicinal plants. He is currently the leading figure in their research committee.

In 1987 as a result of an initiative with a colleague, the University of Exeter set up the Centre for Complementary Health Studies, the first university centre of its type in the developed world. He is one of the two directors of the centre and is responsible for much fascinating research into herbal medicine there.

Simon Mills has been a regular teacher on herbal medicine in the UK and in the USA, for many years making regular flights to New York to maintain a course there. He is also an author of a number of books and articles, including: *The Dictionary of Modern Herbalism*, Thorsons, 1985; (Paperback: *The A-Z of Modern Herbalism* 1989); *Alternatives in Healing*, Macmillan 1988; (Paperback: *Your Health: Your Choice* 1988); *Out of the Earth: The Essential Book of Herbal Medicine*, Viking Penguin 1991.

Foreword

The history of agnus-castus is a long and fascinating one. Since the days of ancient Greece, when the plant was associated with chastity and dedicated to the mother goddess Demeter, it has been used for women's ailments, particularly those connected with menstruation, lactation and the menopause.

In this book Simon Mills tells the story of the use of agnus-castus through the ages, up to the present day. He summarises a number of reports on its action, including a detailed study recently carried out under his direction on the use of agnus-castus for premenstrual tension.

Although we now know much about the chemistry and pharmacology of agnus-castus we still do not yet understand fully how it acts. Without itself having any direct hormonal action it nevertheless gently influences the body's hormonal balance to good effect.

In a chapter describing the menstrual cycle the author gives a lucid account of the bodily and hormonal changes involved (the book could be recommended for this chapter alone). He indicates the ways in which agnus-castus can influence the cycle at different levels. He concludes by describing the complaints and disturbances, not exclusively female, in which agnus-castus may be of help.

This very readable and helpful book is good evidence for the way in which a knowledge of herbs and herbal medicine continues to have an important place in health care today.

Dr John Cosh
MD FRCP

1 | Woman medicine

In the summer heat and sun of the lands and islands of the northern Mediterranean where the olive trees are, there among the wild oleanders with their startling pink flowers, the scrubby tamarisks and the bright green figs, grows an extraordinary tree. It has shrubby growth with long stalks ending in small slender palm-like leaflets, but can reach a height more than twice that of a man. In July and August it produces spikes of lavender-coloured flowers that quickly give way to bunches of seeds the size of peppercorns. The most striking feature however at this stage of late summer is the tree's fragrance.

The fresh flowering, and especially fruiting spikes have a powerful, unique and very evocative pungent, warm and heavy scent. From time immemorial it has been claimed as their own by women.

In Roman times the tree they called *Vitex* was dedicated to the goddess Hera, the protector of motherhood and marriage, who was said to have been born under one. Vestal virgins carried twigs from the tree as a symbol of chastity.

In classical Greece at this time the tree was called αγνος, agnos, meaning holy, pure or chaste. They also dedicated it to their mother goddess, Demeter. At the festival of Thermophona held in her honour, Greek women, whose duty was to remain chaste for the occasion, strewed their beds with branches of the tree, and wore garlands of it in the day, so that the aroma might subdue the ardour of any would-be suitor.

In Homer's Iliad, the tree, referred to as λη γος, lygos, a willow or osier, was seen as a symbol of chastity with the power to ward off evil. Pliny, the Roman writer of the first century, who first recorded the name *Vitex* (from a word meaning to twine, like the willow in wickerwork), refers to its use to maintain chastity and claimed it checked violent sexual desire. His Greek contemporary Discorides may have been speaking only part literally when he said the twigs might fend off wolves!

The full botanical name of this tree today, *Vitex agnus-castus*, was coined as a combination of Greek and Latin, possibly as a result of a translation error. It appears the taxonomist knew his latin better than his Greek. He apparently mistook the Greek αγνος (agnos) for the Latin agnus ("lamb", a word that also survives in a medieval German common name for the plant *Schäffmülle*) and feeling that chastity had to be in there somewhere, put in the Latin word, *castus*, meaning chaste. Agnus-castus, the name now most commonly used for the plant, therefore either means "chaste-chaste" or "chaste lamb"!

The link made in classical times between agnus-castus and chastity was maintained into modern Europe. Common English names for the tree are chasteberry or chastetree; equivalent names are used in German and Dutch. Agnus-castus branches were strewn along the processional way taken by novices entering monasteries, a practice still current in some parts of Italy. In a subtle gender-switch from classical times, the plant was adopted to protect the chastity of monks, earning the common name monk's pepper and a reputation for suppressing "the lusts of the flesh".

It is likely that much of this medieval reputation was simply another example of the adoption by the Christian church of earlier Greek and Roman traditions. Mythological reputations are like that. Even in the 1800's, a French writer Cazin alleged that giving agnus-castus to nuns to improve their chastity might have no such effect, and other writers have referred to stimulating properties in some individuals. As we shall see at the end of Chapter 4, there is real ambiguity about the effects of agnus-castus on the male. Monk's pepper might well deserve its double meaning after all!

Agnus-castus is however much more than a cultural icon. In the folk traditions systematised by Hippocrates in the 4th century BC, agnus-castus was recommended for the treatment of wounds, inflammatory conditions and swellings of the spleen, and also for an "issue of blood" and "for helping the afterbirth to come away." Other authorities in ancient Greece and Rome gave similar advice, Dioscorides adding in the 1st century AD that it was warming and drying in nature. Galen agreeing, added "it also procures milk in women's breasts, it procures their courses ... the docoction of the herb or seeds is very good for the pains of the mother, or inflammations of the parts ..."

In the herbals of 16th and 17th century Europe, which reflected contemporary folk and professional usage, there was general agreement about these points. Individual variations had Lonicerus (1679) recommending agnus-castus as an emmenagogue (promoting menstruation), anaphrodisiac and lactogogue (increasing milk production), and Gerard (1597) suggesting it for the swelling of the genitals and pain and inflammation of the womb. What is known of folk use in countries of the north-eastern Mediterranean has agnus-castus being invariably used for menstrual problems, lower abdominal complaints in general, and to promote milk flow in nursing mothers. These practical folk traditions are the most significant pointer to the real potential of agnus-castus. To see this point however a slight detour in our story is necessary.

Herbs were almost the only medicines available for illnesses and injury in the past. Learning how to use them was often a question of survival. It is apparent from looking at many traditional cultures that most humans used their natural intelligence to good effect and came up with some canny techniques. There were a number of consistently applied approaches for the major priorities of the day: wounds, fevers, intestinal infections, liver disease and lung infections. These were practicable techniques that are often explicable in modern medical terms. *And they were most often applied by women.*

There is a misleading modern image of the "witch-doctor" that sees the traditional healer as often male. As soon as communities became in anyway complex, the uniquely human capacities to imagine, to articulate emotions and to dream lead to a search for wider explanations of illness and misfortune. Individuals able to provide explanations and promote solutions in these terms prospered. They became shamans, "witch-doctors" and eventually, as their work became organised, priests. They often used herbs but mostly in symbolic dream-directed ways. They were most often men.

In reality however if one had a physical ailment in early times one would most likely seek more immediate practical treatment. If it was a job beyond ones own skills, the person one would turn to would most often be a woman, a "wise woman", someone with the knack of using plants for healing. This would practically always be so if the sufferer was a woman or a child. By and large women treated each other. Matters of

CHAP. 54. *Of the Chafte Tree.*

1 *Vitex, five Agnus Caftus.*
The Chafte tree.

‡ 2 *Vitex latiore ferrato folio.*
Chafte tree with cut leaues.

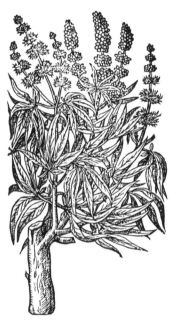

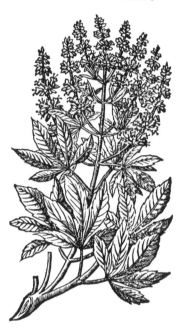

Aaaaaa 2

¶*The*

The above and opposite reproduced from
The Herball or General Historie of Plants *by John Gerard, 1597.*

12

¶ The Defcription.

1   Vitex,or the Chafte tree, groweth after the manner of a bufhie fhrub or hedge tree, hauing many twiggie branches, very pliant and eafie to be bent without breaking, like to the willow:the leaues are for the moft part diuided into fiue or feuen fe&ions or diuifions,much like the leaues of Hemp,whereof each part is long and narrow,very like vnto the willow leafe,but fmaller : the floures do grow at the vppermoft parts of the branches, like vnto fpikie eares,cluftering together about the branches,of a light purple or blew colour,and very fweet fmel: the fruit is fmall and round,like vnto the graines or cornes of pepper.

‡ 2   Lobel mentions another varietie hereof that differs from the former onely in that it hath broader leaues,and thefe alfo fnipt about the edges. ‡

¶ The Place.

Vitex groweth naturally in Italy,and other hot regions,by water courfes and running ftreames: I haue it growing in my garden.

¶ The Time.

Vitex beginneth to recouer his laft leaues in May, and the floures come forth in Auguft.

¶ The Names.

†   The Grecians call this fhrub ἄγνος and λύγος: Agnos(i.) Caſtus,Chafte : becaufe,faith Pliny in his 24.booke,9.Chapter,the Athenian Matrons in their feaft called Thefmophoria dedicated to the honour of Ceres,defirous to keepe themfelues chafte,doe lay the leaues in their beds vnder them : the Latines name it Vitex , and of diuers it is termed,as wee finde among the baftard and counterfeit names,ἄγνος in Latine, Salix marina, or Salix Amerina, and Piper Agrefte : in high Dutch,**Schaff-mulle,Keufchbaum :** in low Dutch,and alfo of the Apothecaries,Agnus Caſtus : the Italians,Vitice, Agno Caſto : in Spanifh,Gattile caſto: in Englifh,Chafte tree,Hempe tree,and of diuers Agnus caſtus. ‡ The name Agnus Caſtus comes by confounding the Greeke name Agnos with Caſtus,the Latine interpretation thereof. ‡

¶ The Temperature.

The leaues and fruit of Agnus caſtus are hot and drie in the third degree : they are of very thin parts,and wafte or confume winde.

The Vertues.

A   Agnus Caſtus is a fingular medicine and remedie for fuch as would willingly liue chafte, for it withftandeth all vncleanneffe,or defire to the flefh, confuming and drying vp the feed of generation, in what fort foeuer it be taken, whether in pouder onely, or the deco&ion drunke, or whether the leaues be carried about the body ; for which caufe it was called Caſtus; that is to fay, chafte, cleane,and pure.

B   The feed of Agnus Caſtus drunken,driueth away, and diffolueth all windineffe of the ftomacke, openeth and cureth the ftoppings of the liuer and fpleen;and in the beginning of dropfies,it is good to be drunke in wine in the quantitie of a dram.

C   The leaues ftamped with butter,diffolue and affwage the fwellings of the genitories and cods, being applied thereto.

D   The deco&ion of the herbe and feed is good againft pain and inflammations about the matrix, if women be caufed to fit and bathe their priuy parts therein : the feed being drunke with Pennyroiall bringeth downe the menfes,as it doth alfo Loth in a fume and in a peffary : in a Pultis it cureth the head-ache,the Phrenticke,and thofe that haue the Lethargie are woont to be bathed herewith,oile and vineger being added thereto.

E   The leaues vfed in a fume,and alfo ftrowed, driue away ferpents ; and beeing layed on doe cure their bitings.

F   The feed laied on with water doth heale the clifts or rifts of the fundament;with the leaues,it is a remedie for lims out of ioint,and for wounds.

G   It is reported that if fuch as iourney or trauell do carry with them a branch or rod of Agnus Caſtus in their hand,it will keep them from Merry-galls,and wearineffe : Diofc.

menstruation and the menstrual cycle, of pregnancy and childbirth, of breastfeeding and child-rearing, were entirely women's work. Men were mostly excluded from this world. Male attendance at childbirth or involvement in infant feeding was extremely rare. Their views of menstruation varied in different cultures from seeing it as a sacred lunar event celebrating fertility, to being a mark of evil, literally a taboo (from the Polynesian *tapoor* a word describing the mystical properties of the menstrual cycle). The actual experience of the women undergoing such events was almost never noted in the early texts, mostly written by men. When Hippocrates, Dioscorides or Galen noted that a remedy was being used for problems of menstruation they were writing about something of which they could have had only a dim and indirect experience.

Women discovered what helped them best to deal with problems of menstruation or childbirth and passed the information on, among themselves. Most has never been written down. Where, as for example, in North America, attempts were made by modern Europeans to record native women's remedies it is clear that these could be sophisticated (and from modern clinical experience with native North American women's remedies such as helonias root, blue cohosh, beth root and squaw vine, also effective).

Europe until the 20th century was as male-dominated a culture as any. Relatively few herbs specifically used by women have survived to figure prominently as such in the modern European herbal materia medica. When a herbal remedy comes to us with an ancient dedication to goddesses of motherhood, then its folk use for women's ailments takes on such a prominence. Although largely neglected by medical authorities until recently (not surprisingly), modern medical research is beginning to indicate that agnus-castus is a very interesting remedy for women indeed.

The story almost certainly starts with a powerful aroma. Whether this has the anaphrodisiac effects claimed may be the subject for further research (although the scent does bring to mind recent discoveries about those strange chemicals, pheromones, that subtly influence libido); it is most likely that much of the plant's association with chastity is symbolic, a cultural, even shamanistic veneer. What we will now concentrate on is the modern potential for the use of agnus-castus by women for a variety of gynaecological and hormone-related problems.

To do this we need first to look at where and how it might work.

2 | The ovarian clock and hormonal balance

The body as powerhouse

It is quite understandable to think of the body as made up of solid parts, like a machine, parts that are simply waiting to go wrong. Modern medical science indeed encourages this view. Just as you go to a mechanic to fix your car, so you go to the doctor to fix the broken parts in your body. If there is nothing obviously wrong with any body parts the assumption is that the problem must therefore "be all in the mind". The body is seen as certainly too complicated to leave to the patient to sort out in anything but the most minor illness.

This is only a very modern view. It was Hippocrates over two thousand years ago who stated firmly that the physician did not heal, that it was the *vis medicatrix naturae*, the healing powers of life itself. The best that a doctor could do was to help healing to occur, at worst he interfered with it.

Modern medicine, for the first three-quarters of the 20th century, began to think it had nailed the Hippocratic idea; modern drugs would finally sort out diseases for good. Now, as we begin to realise they do no such thing, science rediscovers in a number of ways how right Hippocrates was. The body is not just bits and pieces controlled by the brain: the whole, brain included, works as one. The mind is not just up in the head, the body also has a mind of its own, an essential part of the whole.

If this is true for the body as a whole, it is dramatically so for the reproductive organs, especially in women. They remain largely undeveloped until adolescence, developing suddenly at puberty, receding again in later life. In the years between, all the reproductive tissues are involved in a series of cyclic changes, mostly at a lunar interval. These involve considerable alterations to the very structures of ovaries, womb, breasts and their associated tissues. If conception occurs and an embryo implants in the lining of the womb the changes are extraordinary, moving the body through pregnancy and labour, and leading to further changes after birth with the development of milk production from the breasts. *These are changes that compare with any that modern medicine can perform, yet they are entirely self controlled.* They all normally resolve themselves in their allotted time without any outside help.

The primary controlling agents for these dramatic events are the body's hormones. These extremely powerful chemicals are produced from glands such as the ovary, pituitary and adrenal cortex; other even more powerful versions are produced spontaneously from other cells and tissues at the very site. To really understand the potential of agnus-castus it is necessary to learn a little about the way these hormones interact with each other and with the tissues they control. *Everything we know about agnus-castus suggests that it operates at this level.*

The menstrual dance

When one looks at changes that occur for example, in the monthly menstrual cycle, the ways in which the hormones and tissues interact with each other, one can only be impressed by the complexity and delicacy of the choreography. Yet as we go through the sequence it is as well to note that the whole performance is astonishingly robust. In the majority of women the menstrual cycle is rock steady, being barely altered by outside events or other shifts in body functions. This is a key theme in this book: *the body normally runs its affairs very well indeed*; a good medicine might therefore be one that gently nudges it back on track when it becomes disrupted.

There are three main sites where the hormones controlling the menstrual cycle are produced, the ovaries, the pituitary at the base of the brain, and the hypothalamus within the brain itself. The *ovaries* produce mainly "steroidal" hormones, like *oestrogens* (the principal example being βoestradiol), progestins (of which *progesterone* is the dominant example) and androgens (notably *testosterone*). The *pituitary* produces mainly "trophic" hormones that act to switch on hormone production at other sites, like the thyroid, adrenal cortex and testicles in the male: it is for this reason the pituitary is sometimes referred to as the "conductor of the endocrine orchestra". In the following case we will be concerned primarily with two of its hormones, *follicle-stimulating hormone* (FSH) and *luteinising hormone* (LH), although the pituitary also produces *prolactin* and *oxytocin* which are

THE OVARIAN CLOCK

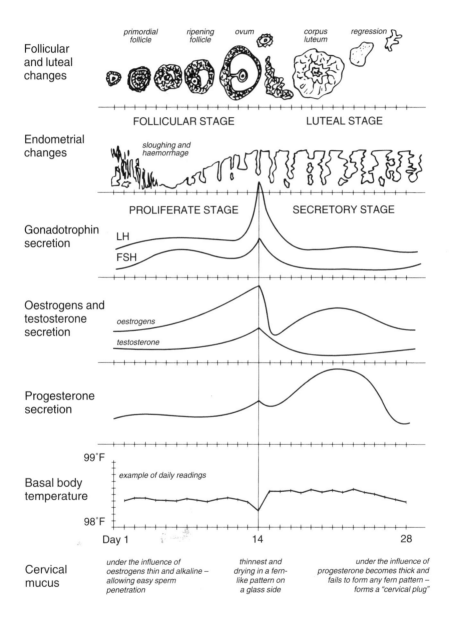

Follicular and luteal changes

primordial follicle | ripening follicle | ovum | corpus luteum | regression

FOLLICULAR STAGE   LUTEAL STAGE

Endometrial changes

sloughing and haemorrhage

PROLIFERATE STAGE   SECRETORY STAGE

Gonadotrophin secretion

LH

FSH

Oestrogens and testosterone secretion

oestrogens

testosterone

Progesterone secretion

Basal body temperature

99°F

example of daily readings

98°F

Day 1   14   28

Cervical mucus

under the influence of oestrogens thin and alkaline – allowing easy sperm penetration

thinnest and drying in a fern-like pattern on a glass side

under the influence of progesterone becomes thick and fails to form any fern pattern – forms a "cervical plug" important in lactation. The pituitary in turn is influenced by a site in the brain itself, the *hypothalamus*, which releases a number of "releasing hormones" to switch on pituitary production. There is one that has been referred to as *luteinising hormone releasing hormone* (LHRH); however as it now appears to facilitate both FSH and LH production it is now often called *gonadotrophin releasing hormone* (GnRH). Although it does not have complete control over pituitary activity the presence of GnRH does provide an opportunity for the brain to influence the menstrual cycle; it also provides a possible mechanism for the action of agnus–castus.

An important point to remember is that each cell that produces a hormone is itself, like all cells in the body, sensitive to the levels of hormones in the fluids around it, and may be partially sensitive to the levels of hormone it itself produces. This is called "negative feedback": it means that as an essential safety feature many hormones switch off their own production. Each hormone may selectively switch on or switch off the production of other hormones as well.

We can start the menstrual sequence at the first day of the period, the end of the previous cycle. The accompanying diagram may make the explanations easier. The pituitary, responding to a sudden drop in steroid hormone levels at the end of the cycle, begins to secrete FSH. This enters the bloodstream and reaches the ovaries. Here its effect is to nudge into activity some of the several hundred thousand *primordial follicles*, each made up of a potential egg or *ovum* and a layer of surrounding cells, that have been sitting in suspended animation in the ovaries since birth. The activated follicles now begin to proliferate, under the continued influence of FSH, with the outer layer beginning to secrete hormones, primarily oestrogens. The follicle that becomes most active by producing more hormones switches off potential activity in other competitor follicles, in both ovaries. These then shrink and the successful candidate becomes the *primary follicle* and grows rapidly. As a result the levels of oestrogens rise in the bloodstream. The oestrogens have a number of effects in the body: their first job is to prepare a new womb lining, promoting the growth of new nutrient-rich mucosa, but also preparing the Fallopian tubes and the vaginal epithelium for possible eventual conception. They also tend to raise metabolic rate and blood sugar levels and to have a stimulating effect; the woman is likely to feel more alert and decisive.

As the follicle develops, a process lasting approximately 10 days, the levels of oestrogens in the blood rise higher, and androgens like testosterone also begin to increase (these will tend to increase libido). All this begins to depress further FSH production and encourages the pituitary instead to begin secretion of LH. As the follicle ripens the levels of oestrogens become so high that they trigger a crescendo effect, in a process sometimes explained as "positive feedback", where high levels of hormone encourage more rather than less production. There are sudden surges, first in oestrogen, and then dramatically in LH production and lesser peaks in FSH and testosterone. The effect is to rupture the ripe follicle and release the ovum to be drawn by an activated Fallopian tube lining, down towards the womb already primed for possible implantation. This ends the first, *follicular* stage of the menstrual cycle.

The surge in LH, probably the critical factor in ovulation, also switches off most oestrogen production and converts the cells of the remnant follicle to producing a new set of steroid hormones, including new oestrogens but notably progesterone. This remnant also changes shape and colour to become the *corpus luteum*, meaning "yellow body". The corpus luteum grows under the influence of LH for about 10 days through the second *luteal* half of the cycle, unless conception and implantation occur, in which case new hormones are produced from the implant to maintain it for up to three weeks, until its function can be taken over by the placenta. The progesterone it produces starts by enriching the womb lining and in similar ways creating the optimum environment in the womb for the start of pregnancy. Progesterone also switches off LH production, reducing contractions in the womb and Fallopian tubes, and generally has a calming effect on the body. Women at this stage can feel generally more relaxed, although this can be diminished as oestrogen levels may often also be high.

If no conception occurs the corpus luteum runs out of hormone-producing capacity after about 10 days. Levels of both progesterone and oestrogens begin to fall. The corpus luteum therefore has the job both of maintaining the second half of the menstrual cycle and of ensuring a clean menstruation. It is worth noting at this point *that all clinical experience and research points to agnus-castus having as its main effect the support of the corpus luteum.*

The whole menstrual cycle can therefore be seen as the result of a subtle interplay of hormones with each other, through negative and positive feedback, and with the tissues they affect. The rate-determining agent is the cells in the ovary. The time taken for the follicle to develop, new hormones to be produced, and ovulation to be possible is not easily altered. The life-span of the corpus luteum is also largely its own affair. The length of the cycle and of its stages is therefore set by the development of the primordial follicle in the ovary – it has sometimes been referred to as the "ovarian clock".

Conception and beyond

Let us now turn briefly to the hormonal events that lead into pregnancy. If conception occurs the events of the follicular half of the cycle will have ensured the optimum environment for the ruptured fertilised egg. It would be wafted down the Fallopian tube by activated fronds, or *cilia*, with nourishing fluids secreted from the walls. After fertilisation by the sperm, usually somewhere along the tube, it should then reach the uterus to land somewhere on a mucosal-lining, spongy-rich with blood supply and nourishment. The conceptus will have already been multiplying to form an outer wall of cells to protect the developing embryo. This wall will secrete enzymes that allow it to burrow deep into the mucosa – *implantation* will then have occurred; it will also be secreting new hormones to support the corpus luteum for an extra ten days or so after its natural lifespan. In that time part of the embryo's protecting outer wall will have proliferated to become the *placenta*, burrowing into more of the womb lining to set up the all-important connection with the mother's circulation. The placenta itself becomes a major hormone producer and largely takes over control of the pregnancy. As every mother knows the changes in her body at this time are astonishing – from the womb increasing in size some twentyfold, the heart increasing production by 30–40%, the metabolic rate by 15%, the ligaments of the pelvis softening, the breasts developing and enlarging, as well as considerable emotional shifts. Almost all these changes are the result of increasing levels of the main reproductive hormones, produced by the placenta, ovary and adrenal cortex. After a while the baby's own glands contribute hormonal influences, and labour itself is brought on by a burst of hormones from the baby; it really does know when it wants to come out!

With the birth and the loss of the placenta there is another substantial hormonal shift – one that in a few cases can be very traumatic to the mother – before the ovaries and the pituitary pick up a new rhythm. Here progesterone provides the bass note, with the lead taken over by another pituitary hormone, prolactin. Together they lead to milk production by the glandular tissues in the breast *(this is another area where agnus-castus has a strong traditional reputation)*. The "letting down" of milk at feed is induced by a new short-term pituitary hormone, oxytocin, that incidentally helps with the recovery of the womb and other structures after the pregnancy.

Hormones – gentle giants

This account of pregnancy and lactation reiterates again the extraordinary power of hormones. These include determining our very emotions. It is theoretically possible to recreate many emotional feelings by injecting the right cocktail of hormones. Adrenaline produces arousal and anxiety, insulin is euphoric, testosterone produces aggression and increased libido, the adrenal steroids are calming, and we have already seen the main effects of the female sex hormones. This may sound alarming and even mechanical – *"you mean all my feelings are determined by chemicals?"* In fact they only provide the foundations, other circumstances provide the fine tuning. More importantly however, hormones are not tyrants. We have seen that they generally do what they are supposed to do, and then stop. They are simply agents, powerful agents it is true, of the whole body. If they reproduce fear, anxiety, depression, temper tantrums, joy, or even mad manic delight, well, something has to! If these emotional symptoms become persistent or troublesome it is rarely the fault of the hormones. Their job is to integrate the body and mind and their many facets into one whole being and enable that to adapt to the demands of the environment. If they are causing trouble then they usually mean that something else is wrong.

All this is most relevant to the story of agnus-castus. This herb is most likely to interact with a woman's hormones. We will see that this has implications not only for physical symptoms but for how the woman feels as well.

21

The delicacy of the body's hormonal balance and its emotional consequences are next most apparent to a woman at the time of her menopause, when the menstrual cycles begin to run down.

Hormonal changes

The problem of *menopause* must not be exaggerated. For many women there are simply none. From what we can glean of other cultures and other times it was barely a problem there either. There is no physiological reason why this phase needs to be uncomfortable. Nevertheless for an appreciable number of modern women discomfort is too mild a term for what they have to endure. The almost miraculous properties of artificially administered hormones, hormone replacement therapy (HRT), is an effective indication of how central hormones are to the physical and mental symptoms of a troublesome menopause. We will return to this subject again. Enough to note that it would be valuable to have a medicine that helped the body make its own hormonal adjustments if necessary, rather than having to rely on artificial props. *Agnus-castus, though containing no hormones itself, has a strong reputation for helping women through the menopause.*

There is one other life stage when the effect of reproductive hormones is dominant, the time of course when they first emerge as major players, at *puberty*. The changes the body undergoes in adolescence are all very familiar, as are the potential problems of that age. In girls early periods can be erratic and painful as the menstrual rhythm and ovarian clock is set up; in a few this phase can last into adulthood.

Another problem area, in both girls and boys, is the skin. Uneven mixes of the reproductive hormones, especially excessive amounts of the androgens like testosterone, can stimulate the sebaceous glands in the upper part of the body (that normally provide weather protection to the most exposed body surfaces) to over production of sebum. This also more readily clots, causing trouble by blocking the glands' openings, producing a come-do (whitehead or blackhead). Bacterial infection behind these plugs leads to the familiar spots of *acne*. Although agnus-castus has not generally been used for problems of puberty a beneficial effect in the treatment of acne has been noted. A progesteronal action may be significant here.

★　　★　　★

The purpose of this section has been to provide a framework in which to judge the potential of agnus-castus. The emphasis has not only been on the potency of the hormonal regulators of changes in the reproductive system, but also on the message that powerful as they are they still meekly do what they are told. The body can and does control them and directs them to its wider aims. Modern medicine, particularly as it concerns itself with illnesses in women, is prone to forget this. It sees each event in a woman's reproductive life in the same mechanical terms that it sees everything else. If there is a hormonal problem, give artificial hormones. If there is a pregnancy, take the mother to hospital; if the labour does not fit immediate expectations, induce and/or do a Caesarian section. Epidurals, episiotomies, hysterectomies, and mastectomies are all valid and sometimes vital medical manoeuvres, that women sometimes feel can be used too readily.

In the past women tackled many of their problems with their own gentle treatments, treatments that seemed to work with the body on its own terms. In the next chapter we will look at how one such treatment, agnus-castus, might be used in such a way today.

3 | Agnus-castus in modern medicine

Agnus-castus is one of a great many medicinal plants where science has not caught up with popular reputation. The evidence in modern literature for the effect of agnus-castus is made up mostly of clinical observations with few good clinical trials. Nevertheless, taken altogether, a strong circumstantial case is clear, and it is possible to draw some consistent themes from it. It is also possible, in the next chapter, to make specific suggestions as to how it may be applied today.

Let us start with the modern medicine. This derives in large part from Germany. Agnus-castus was rediscovered there in the 1930's and developed into a proprietary formulation by a leading herbal manufacturer in Germany, which resulted in some of the following research.

The chemistry

Some work has been done in attempting to isolate the constituents. The first conclusion has been that agnus-castus does not contain any hormones or anything similar. One is therefore in using this remedy not taking a "natural HRT". The most likely active chemical constituents appear to be:

a group of phenolic compounds called flavonoids (notably casticin, unique to this plant);

terpenoid compounds in the aromatic volatile oil (such as pinene, sabinene, cineole, as well as sesquiterpenes);

iridoids, terpenoid derivatives, such as agnuside and aucubin.

The potential properties of these constituents, or indeed whether they are linked to the properties of the whole plant at all, have not been elucidated. However, they do come from active groups of chemicals and it is quite likely that their effect is significant.

The pharmacology

As already stated agnus-castus does not contain hormones. German pharmacological investigations in the 1940's and 1950's however, indicate that it does induce hormonal changes in the body. The firm conclusion of these early investigators was that the effect of agnus-castus was to promote LH activity in the pituitary and thus to increase corpus luteum activity and, in particular, the secretions of progesterone (see previous chapter). More recent work might now suggest that the hypothalamic GnRH should also be included in this frame. In recent times this scenario has been confirmed and clinical evidence has also tended to support such an idea.

Observations on breastfeeding

Progesterone is a contributor to milk production in lactating mothers. The first recorded clinical observations were on this aspect of the popular reputation of agnus-castus. A number of physicians noted benefits in helping improve problems of breastfeeding. In 1953 a Doctor Bautze showed that among 200 lactating women taking agnus-castus there was increased milk and freer flow than in an equivalent 100 not being treated. Two years later Doctor Mohr compared the breastfeeding performance of 353 women taking agnus-castus with 102 taking vitamin B1, as well as a number of untreated controls. Again there were significant benefits for the group taking agnus-castus. Mohr noted that these were only apparent after two weeks of treatment.

Effects on menstrual problems

Effects of agnus-castus on menstrual disturbances in women are also reported from the mid-1950's. In 1954 for example there were published two observational studies on the effects of taking agnus-castus. In one, physicians Probst and Roth showed beneficial effects, as measured by improvements in cyclic body temperature shifts and in the tissues of womb lining and vaginal wall, in a number of women suffering from secondary amenorrhoea (where the periods stop), from excessive menstrual bleeding, from infertility due to lack of ovulation, or from ovarian cysts. Regular periods were achieved in 50 out of 57 women being observed.

The other report of that year, by Kayser and Istanbulluoglu, showed that taken over the long term the effects of agnus-castus were maintained. Out of their group of 51 women suffering excessive and frequent menstrual bleeding, 33 got good results. They noted that there was seldom any effect before ten days and the best results were observed after six months.

The published literature had only minor or unsupported citations for the next 30 years. From the late 1980's however there have been a number of further studies. In 1988 a team treated 48 women suffering infertility associated with low progesterone levels in the second part of the cycle but who were otherwise normal. After taking agnus-castus 25 women achieved normal progesterone levels and 15 actually became pregnant. A total of 39 women had some change, including lengthening shortened menstrual cycles.

In 1990 two physicians, Loch and Kaiser, treating loss of periods, found that over six and twelve month periods agnus-castus raised progesterone and LH levels, but did not affect, or slightly decreased, FSH levels.

At the same time as these studies were being undertaken a large multi-centre trial was being conducted observing the effects of agnus-castus on 1571 women with a number of menstrual disturbances. Premenstrual syndrome was the most common symptom, with 867 sufferers, and corpus luteum insufficiency was identified in 1318. Treatment time varied from days to many months, but averaged in excess of four months. From a large number of reports from both patients and physicians impressive improvements over a wide range of symptoms were reported, with nearly 90% of total symptoms among the group improved.

The other significant trial from Germany was done in 1968 with acne. There have been several clinical reports published on agnus-castus in this condition and in 1968 Doctors Giss and Rothenburg treated 118 patients of both sexes with acne, comparing their performance to 43 controls. They reported 70% of treated patients had been cured of their acne in three months.

The double-blind clinical trial

These clinical observations make an impressive case for taking agnus-castus, and we shall return to the practical implications of these findings in the next chapter. We must turn briefly however to the requirements of science. The problem so far is that none of these studies were "blinded" clinical trials, and only three had any control group of any sort. To the sceptic who wants proof, it is not enough that people who take agnus-castus get better. It is pointed out a) that things get better of their own accord, b) that good effects can happen by chance, and c) that if you expect things to get better the body is actually likely to make it so. To rule out the first possibility one should have a *control group* of similar sufferers who do not receive treatment and who are watched under similar conditions so their fate can be compared with the treatment group. It is possible to dispense with this if the condition is very longstanding in nature or if one knows enough about it to predict natural change over the time concerned. The trial on infertility might have been able to dispense with a control group for this reason but even here spontaneous recovery of fertility is known.

To minimise the second possible problem one needs to have *sufficient numbers* of similar subjects to reduce the probability that the effects one sees may have happened by chance. The numbers necessary require careful calculation by a statistician.

The third potential distortion in the results is more fundamental. The *placebo effect* (literally: *I please*) is a well-known phenomenon in medicine. It is accepted that if either the patient, or the doctor, expect a medicine to work, then it is much more likely to do so. This is of course particularly so if there is an emotional component to the problem, but placebo cures are known in any disease. This need not be surprising. In fact, from what was described in the previous chapter, one can see that with the enormous self-correcting power of the body, ***most*** healing is of the placebo variety. If you get a cut, it heals itself; so do most things. If the mind and body are one then willing something better is bound to have a good effect. If 80% of patients get better when they have a certain treatment does it matter how much of it the body did on its own? For the sufferer, and perhaps most readers of this book, the answer is that it does not. However those whose job it is to assess medicines need some idea of what they do as far as possible, independently of the body's own contribution. This is very difficult to determine and imposes most unnatural conditions on the treatment. In practice both the patient and the doctor must be unaware whether the treatment being prescribed is the real thing or a dummy placebo, this is the *double-blind clinical trial*.

British research

In the UK such requirements are almost mandatory for those researching herbal remedies. The ability of German physicians to publish non-controlled, non-blinded and unsupported clinical observations on herbal remedies in the scientific literature is a luxury not available in Britain, as medical orthodoxy is much more sceptical. Thus when Gerard House, the British herbal medicine company, introduced agnus-castus to the public it went straight for rigorous trials to assess its potential. The first in 1987 was a pilot on relatively small numbers of women suffering premenstrual syndrome, but with a control group and double-blinding. This showed promising results in the relief of these symptoms.

The second trial was much bigger and more stringent, in fact ruthlessly so. Our team at Exeter University in association with Gerard House, lead by statistician Susan Turner, set out to investigate further properties of agnus-castus in the treatment of premenstrual syndrome. The design was extremely thorough to counter any possible accusation of bias. Over 2300 women readers of a popular newspaper and a magazine were recruited for the project. We chose 600 who had a suitable range of symptoms and then randomly assigned them to two equal matched groups (to avoid the risk that there might be bias or distortion in the selection). The earlier study, as well as later market research that year, had suggested that the main effect of agnus-castus was on the emotional symptoms of PMS. We therefore used a standard questionnaire that had been tried and tested to accurately register such changes, and then set exact criteria by which we wished to measure improvement.

The results were very interesting. At the time of writing they await formal review and a decision about whether to publish or proceed with further trials, so exact details cannot yet be produced. However they confirmed a high response to placebo for this condition. Over half those taking the dummy pills showed substantial improvements in their symptoms. In fact although there was some advantage with agnus-castus it was impossible to say statistically that it had a significant effect (i.e. an effect that was not due to chance) on the emotional symptoms of PMS over and above that of the placebo.

However, with another symptom of PMS, fluid retention and breast tenderness, there was a suggestion of a significant advantage. Unfortunately we had not set out the measures to monitor these symptoms and were thus unable to show such a result conclusively. This may be the subject of an other study, but even the result we had, given the stringency of the trial design, does more to point to a real benefit for users of agnus-castus in scientific circles than do other apparently more impressive results that were nôt controlled.

During the trial the research team invited additional comments from subjects. About half included various comments on the treatment with their returned questionnaires. At the time they came in of course, because of the double-blind nature of the trial, the research team was unable to say whether the senders were taking agnus-castus or not. However after the trial, when the code was broken, we were surprised to see that over five times as many positive comments were received from women taking agnus-castus than from those receiving the placebo. Such findings were impossible to formally assess but they do reinforce the experience that agnus-castus can have dramatic benefits.

The placebo effect we found is interesting. We had reinforced an obvious point: emotionally-related problems are most easily corrected by positive thoughts and expectations. Our group suffered to the extent that they had been told they might be taking a placebo – it is no wonder that improvement levels were less than in non-blinded trials.

This reminds us again of the link between hormones and emotions. In this sort of trouble it is in fact impossible to disentangle which produces what. If one is encouraged to feel better about ones illness that actually changes hormonal activity itself. If hormones are central to the problem this really does mean that positive expectations can literally and directly correct it. It is even possible, as we have seen, that agnus-castus might work at the level of the hypothalamus, the part of the brain responsible for co-ordinating mental and emotional activities with internal body functions. If this was the case one can see that this would be a herb one could never be able to take impartially!

This all makes clinical research more difficult. In due course new trials should investigate further the non-emotionally mediated effects of agnus-castus, to quantify exactly how it works. In the meantime there is an undeniably strong clinical and personal record to back up its ancient tradition. The evidence has been enough to convince the government authorities in Germany. In the official Government monograph for agnus-castus (*Bundesanzeiger Nummer 90, vomn 15,05,85*) the following headings, below, appear (with translation):

Anwendungsgebeite	Indications
Menstruationsstörungen infolge primärer und sekundärer Gelbkörperinsuffizienz. Prämenstruelles Syndrom. Mastodynie, klimakterische Beschwerden, mangelhafte Stilleistung.	Menstrual disorders following primary or secondary corpus luteum insufficiency. Premenstrual syndrome, breast inflammations, menopausal symptoms and poor lactation.

Gegenanzeigen	Contra-indications
Keine bekannt.	None known.

Nebenwirkungen	Side-effects
In seltenen Fällen zu frühe Wiederkehr der Periode nach der Geburt (Hypophysenaktivierung). Gelegentliches Auftreten von juckenden, urtikariellen Exanthemen.	It occasionally causes menstruation to start earlier after childbirth (due to activation of the pituitary). It can induce occasional itching and urticaria.

Wechselwirkungen	Interaction with other drugs
Keine bekannt.	None known.

4 | Agnus-castus: the clinical potential

In this chapter we will review the modern experience of agnus-castus in more detail. We will combine this with some theoretical information and what is thought about the effects of agnus-castus on the body. It will be useful to refer back to Chapter 2 for elucidation on this.

Before we go any further a strong caution must be sounded. What follows are clinical recommendations for the use of agnus-castus, as would be made to qualified medical herbalists or interested physicians, as well as a few suggestions about when not to use it. Self-treatment always carries more risks. Illness can be unpredictable even when it looks straight-forward; simple symptoms may hide dangerous disease. Before any reader seeks to use agnus-castus on her own account she should be satisfied of the following:

a) she has had her symptoms thoroughly assessed by her doctor and if possible one qualified as a gynaecologist or obstetrician (the letters DRCOG or DObst after a doctor's name denote such training) or a consultant, and she reports any new symptom. Particular "red-flag' symptoms are:

any bleeding outside the expected period, unusual pains in the pelvic area or on intercourse, vaginal discharge, especially if malodorous, and any lump or obstruction;

b) she is not also taking powerful prescription drugs, notably "blood-thinning" (i.e. anticoagulant) drugs, digoxin, insulin, or anti-epileptics;

c) she should not be pregnant (see below).

Although not contra-indicated, taking the Pill, HRT, or other hormonal medication may reduce the effects of agnus-castus in some cases.

It is also worth emphasising that if one is taking the self-medication route one should take all the other responsibilities that entails. Routine self-examination of breasts and checking vaginal discharges and other signs is still the best way to spot any trouble before it becomes serious.

In pursuing any herbal route it may also be worth consulting a practitioner expert in these matters. Qualified medical herbalists, members of the National Institute of Medical Herbalists, with the letters MNIMH or FNIMH after their name will have received four years training in the clinical application of herbal remedies for a wide range of problems and will be able to make a balanced judgement about their use. They will all be familiar with agnus-castus.

Even with such precautions the unexpected can always happen, and as stated in the Note to Reader, no liability can be accepted by the author if the reader chooses to go ahead with self-treatment.

Having made that point it is also fair to reiterate that agnus-castus has an excellent safety record. No serious adverse effects are expected.

Let us start by seeing how agnus-castus may lend itself to the correction of menstrual disorders. A reminder first: agnus-castus does not contain hormones and is unlikely therefore to force any changes. Clinical experience suggests that it interacts with the body's own hormonal balance in some way, possibly by affecting the hypothalamus (GnRH) – pituitary (LH) – corpus luteum (progesterone) axis. It is gentle in action, nudging self-correction rather than working unilaterally, and it needs to be taken for some weeks before any effect is likely. In treating a menstrual disorder a medical herbalist would generally allow a minimum of three months for significant changes to have had time to take place.

Irregular or frequent periods

These can occur with any disruption of the "ovarian-clock", either in the follicular or luteal phase or both. Clinical experience suggests agnus-castus is more suited to the latter. The best way to establish what is happening is to use a basal body temperature chart to find when, or if, ovulation has occurred. A basal body temperature chart can be obtained by recording everyday your temperature, using a conventional clinical thermometer in the mouth, immediately on waking and before doing anything else. Taken over the month there is typically a rise of around half a degree Centigrade at ovulation maintained more or less for the second part of the month. If ovulation precedes menstruation by about 14 days then the corpus luteum is probably in working order and agnus-castus may not be so useful. If however this luteal phase is short, as it often is, or if the pattern is not at all clear, then agnus castus is worth a trial.

Absent periods (amenorrhoea)

If the start of periods at puberty is delayed this is technically referred to as *primary amenorrhoea*. Sometimes this merits expert examination. However the great majority of cases sort themselves out in time and no treatment is usually justified. If existing periods stop then that is referred to as *secondary amenorrhoea*. By far the main cause is pregnancy and this must be excluded before treatment is applied. Some plants were indeed used by women to "promote menstruation" (i.e. they were used as abortifacients and have since been termed *emmenagogues*). Agnus-castus is not one of them. If however loss of periods occurs without pregnancy and there is not another organic cause, then agnus-castus has a clinical reputation for bringing them back in some cases. Treatment may have to be extended for up to a year and check-ups should be taken during that time.

Heavy periods (menorrhagia)

These can occur for a number of reasons. Fibroids or other mechanical obstructions or inflammations should be checked for. Agnus-castus is most likely to benefit heavy periods that are preceded by a phase of congestion (see also PMS opposite) but may be useful in other non-complicated cases.

Painful periods (dysmenorrhoea)

These commonly occur in the early periods of adolescence, typically as spasms during menstruation itself. This form sometimes termed *spasmodic* or *primary dysmenorrhoea*, is caused by spasm of the womb blood vessels (similar to angina in the heart) and usually passes in the first pregnancy. It has occasionally been treated by dilatation of the womb for the same reason. There is no particular evidence that agnus-castus has benefit here but it would not be ruled out.

It is certainly indicated for another type of painful period – *congestive dysmenorrhoea* – that arises in the days preceding menstruation and may be relieved by the period itself. This type can be seen perhaps as an extension of the same disorders that lead to premenstrual syndrome, discussed next.

⚕ Painful periods may also follow inflammatory disease in the pelvic area, ovarian cysts or endometriosis (see page 36). These possibilities should be excluded in any case.

Premenstrual syndrome (PMS)

Many women suffer a range of symptoms in the days preceding their periods. There are many variations reported. One classification system groups symptoms into four categories, although in fact many women suffer from more than one:

PMT-A: irritability, nervous tension, mood swings, anxiety.

PMT-H: fluid retention, breast tenderness, abdominal bloating, weight gain.

PMT-C: sweet or chocolate cravings, increased appetite, headache, palpitations, fatigue, light-headedness.

PMT-D: depression, crying, confusion, forgetfulness, insomnia.

Relative deficiencies of corpus luteum function and progesterone levels have been implicated as causes of at least some PMS symptoms, although other hormonal disturbances have also been suggested. Other types of menstrual trouble marked by a build-up of symptoms before the period, such as congestive dysmenorrhoea or heavy periods after premenstrual congestion should probably be considered as aspects of PMS. From the results of the Exeter clinical trial it might be expected that agnus–castus would be most suitable for category PMT-H above, and for other problems marked by fluid retention and congestion. However a great number of PMS sufferers of all types experience benefit from agnus–castus (it remains the main reason for spontaneous testimonials from grateful women) and the first, albeit small British double-blind clinical study showed good results in categories PMT-A and PMT-D as well as PMT-H. Given its safety and the lack of other medical interest in the syndrome, then anyone with this problem might try agnus–castus.

Infertility

Inability to conceive can arise from a wide variety of reasons not all of course to do with the woman. Those that are not due to problems with the sperm or the woman's compatibility with it can be broadly divided into two groups: those due to structural or mechanical problems (like blockage of the Fallopian tubes or ovarian damage), and the majority due to functional problems. The latter include the inability of the ovarian clock to perform on cue (often marked by a disturbed menstrual cycle) or problems in implanting in the womb lining. Hormone production or tissue response to hormones may also be inadequate.

The report in 1988 of the relative success of agnus-castus where infertility was associated with low progesterone counts shows it is certainly worth trying at least in this case. It could be considered in fact in any case where infertility is judged to be due to a functional disorder, although probably not worth taking beyond six months, unless hormonal counts or other measures (for example an improved menstrual cycle) were seen to be moving well.

★   ★   ★

So far we have considered *symptoms* of menstrual trouble, most often referring to *functional* disorders, i.e. those produced by errant behaviour of the parts concerned. More *organic* damage is generally considered inappropriate for non-expert treatment. However many gynaecological problems are poorly treated in conventional terms, and apart from surgery are often left untreated. Women can suffer them for many years. The following sections therefore refer both to the advisability of taking agnus-castus at all, and also to the prospects that it may even be of benefit. The assumption is obviously that all the following have been thoroughly assessed by expert medical opinion and that clearance has been given to go ahead with agnus-castus treatment.

Fibroids

These are very common in women but are also of mysterious origin. They are most often harmless but can provoke heavy bleeding at menstruation and can occasionally cause enough trouble for a hysterectomy to be considered. Many women with fibroids have taken agnus-castus and have claimed relief from such symptoms and there have been no reports of their exacerbation. Reports of fibroids shrinking defeat current medical explanation.

Ovarian cysts

Fluid-filled cysts in the ovaries are also quite common. Some are permanent and need closer examination to make sure they are benign or not causing hormonal problems in their own right. Removal of an ovary may rarely be necessary. Most cysts are however "functional", being in fact exaggerated follicles or corpus lutea. These develop and recede in line with the particular phase of the month. A *follicular cyst* will be apparent (on palpation or in some other way) in the first half of the menstrual cycle and will recede at ovulation. A *luteal cyst* will become so after ovulation and recede at menstruation. Either can lead to, be accompanied by, or even cause hormonal disruption, that in turn can lead to any of the other menstrual symptoms discussed above.

Agnus-castus may be inappropriate for treating luteal cysts, possibly even exaggerating them, but it may be helpful with follicular cysts. *In most cases though caution is necessary*.

Pelvic inflammatory disease

Chronic inflammation of the womb (*endometritis*), Fallopian tubes (*salpingitis*) or ovaries (*öophoritis*) and associated structures is an increasingly common condition that follows trauma to these tissues, like infection, abortion or even the coil. It produces pain (especially on deep penetration, and at ovulation – *Mittelschmerz*), pelvic congestion, heavy and painful periods, and/or discharges. It proves resistant to antibiotic and other conventional treatments and there is a potential risk of infertility if left altogether. Herbal practitioners have often seen good results in treating the problem.

There is no recent anti-inflammatory reputation for agnus–castus (although an ancient one – see the first chapter) and it is less likely that it would sort out this condition on its own. However it often features in herbal prescriptions made up for affected patients, and is very unlikely to cause problems if taken alone.

Endometriosis

This refers to the proliferation of the specialised womb lining in parts of the pelvic cavity outside the uterus. It causes symptoms often indistinguishable from pelvic inflammatory disease. There are a number of possible causes but few ways to treat it short of surgery, itself often difficult.

Agnus-castus may in theory have a short-term exacerbatory effect in the luteal phase of the menstrual cycle, but this has not been reported. It is unlikely to alter the condition substantially, however it is recommended by the *Endometriosis Society* in Britain as a treatment for its members and it may be effective in reducing some symptoms.

We can now look at other conditions and review the potential of agnus-castus in these cases.

Pregnancy

Agnus-castus is not specifically ruled out in pregnancy and no particular problems have ever been reported. Nevertheless its ability to interact with key hormonal controls prompts caution in its use here. The simple message should be: ***when pregnant do not take anything that is not essential***. Agnus-castus has no reputation for treating problems of pregnancy and should be discontinued as soon as pregnancy is confirmed.

Breastfeeding

Improving milk flow in lactating mothers is probably the most persistent traditional use of agnus-castus. As progesterone is a key player in setting up lactation this can be readily accepted, although it is also quite possible that other hormonal interactions might be involved as well. There seems little reason to discourage use of the herb during breastfeeding. Transfer of the herb's constituents through the breast milk is likely to be minimal and there is little reason to suspect their influence on the infant anyway (the effect on adults presumes an active reproductive system). The clinical research referred to in the last chapter noted that there were few results before two weeks.

Menopausal problems

Agnus-castus has in its recent use been strongly favoured for the treatment of all menopausal problems, whether hot flushes, fluid retention, emotional disturbances or depression. Some women report effects from taking agnus-castus comparable to those of HRT. Replacement with synthetic hormones has been seen by many as a harmless boost to women suffering menopausal symptoms. However it has begun to raise real doubts in some clinicians and one team has published in *The Lancet* their observations of HRT prescribing and its effects on women, comparing it to the prescription of addictive drugs like cocaine. Those concerned that the body should on the whole sort its own problems out would in any case be less than happy with the use of artificial props.

There is every reason to encourage a trial of agnus-castus instead, although there may need to be some delicate readjustment necessary if HRT is already being taken. At least three months of treatment should be allowed to check its effect properly. Its use would accord well with a traditional approach to the treatment of menopausal-type symptoms. Where these are reported at all in ancient texts they are seen as marks of debility and treated with tonic medicines, rest and other convalescent strategies. There is every reason, even now the hormonal mechanisms are better understood, to comply with this ancient advice, and agnus-castus fits very well into a broader supportive traditional strategy.

Acne

This is one case where agnus-castus has been recommended more widely, than for female problems. Experience of the effects of agnus-castus in acne is limited in Britain but there are good clinical observations from Germany. It would seem prudent to limit its trial period to three months if it does not improve symptoms and in girls to note any changes in the menstrual cycles. Boys are unlikely to be adversely affected by taking agnus-castus for a few months, but particular attention should be paid to their responses (see below).

Other conditions

There have been occasional clinical reports of other uses for agnus-castus. The Hippocratic recommendations that it be used for "swellings of the spleen" (actually a clinical effect of liver disease), wounds and inflammatory conditions have not been checked in modern times. These are simply enticing problems for further investigation.

There have been reports of agnus-castus being effective in the treatment of the symptoms of the herpes virus, like cold sores and genital blisters (herpes simplex) and shingles (herpes zoster). Traditional herbal approaches to this problem have been to use "nerve tonics" and convalescent strategies. If agnus-castus did have a role in this area it would be very interesting indeed.

Agnus-castus for men

The ancient writers did not specify that agnus-castus was meant for women only. Many of the original recommendations, like those of Hippocrates above, or of Galen using it "to resist the bitings of venomous beasts" or because it "dissolveth the wind in the stomach or belly being fresh" were made to both sexes alike. There are however probably few pressing reasons why such claims should prompt men or women to try agnus-castus themselves except for those conditions already elaborated in previous pages.

The only substantial modern use recommended to men is the treatment of acne. The question then arises as to what might be the impact on males of taking a herb which was after all traditionally recommended "to restraineth also the instigations to venery" (Galen). One might expect a certain resistance on the part of most men to voluntarily taking a remedy which might subdue their libido! The question is, would such concerns be justified?

As mentioned in the first chapter, it was the *aroma* that was claimed to reduce male ardour rather than taking the plant as a medicine, and there were already doubts even in earlier times that agnus-castus had quite the effect on chastity that the myth suggested. There is also the intriguing point that the hormonal controls in men are quite different from those in women.

We can recall that agnus-castus is thought to act somewhere on the hormonal links between the hypothalamus (GnRH), the pituitary (LH) and the corpus luteum (progesterone). In men however, the effects of LH are to lead to the production not of progesterone, but of *testosterone* from the testes, a hormone with quite the opposite effect on chaste thoughts. If the action of agnus-castus is in anyway weighted towards the pituitary or hypothalamus, then the effects of agnus-castus in men might be the exact opposite to that in women!

In practice there seems to be little reason in fact to expect any effect on venerous attitudes. On the other hand there is sufficiently little modern experience of its effect on men that the recommendation for them must be to use it with care.

5 | Source and dosage

Agnus-castus is available in Britain at all health stores and many pharmacies. It may also be prescribed by medical herbalists either as powdered herb or in the form of an alcoholic tincture.

The dose of agnus-castus is as recommended by the manufacturer. This reflects clinical usage among medical herbalists, and provides adequate quantities for all likely requirements. It is unlikely that this dose would ever need to be exceeded.

Further reading
Böhnert K, -J, and Hahn G, (1990). Phytotherapie in Gynäkologie und Geburtshilfe: Vitex agnus-castus (Keuschlamm): Eine alte Kultur- und Arzneipflanze, Erfahrungsheilkunde, 39, 494-502.

6 | Index

A

abortifacients 35
abortion 38
absent periods
    see *amenorrhoea*
acne 22, 27, 40, 41
adolescents 40
adrenal cortex 16, 20
agnos 9
agnuside 25
"all in the mind" 15
amenorrhoea 26, 35
androgens 16, 19, 22
anxiety 21, 36
appetite, increased 36
aroma 9, 41
aucubin 25

B

birth 16, 18, 21
bleeding 26, 27, 33, 37
bloating 36
blood sugar 18
breast 21, 39
breast tenderness 29, 36
breastfeeding 14, 26, 39
British research 29

C

casticin 25
caution 33, 38, 39
chasteberry 10
chastetree 10
chastity 9, 10, 14, 41
chemistry 25
chocolate cravings 36
cineole 25
coil, the 38
cold sores 40
conception 15, 18, 19, 20

confusion 36
constituents 25, 39
corpus luteum 17, 19, 20, 25, 31, 34, 36, 41
corpus luteum insufficiency 27, 31
crying 36

D

Demeter 9
depression 21, 36, 39
digoxin 33
Dioscorides 10, 14
double-blind clinical trial 27
drugs 15, 33, 40
dysmenorrhoea 35, 36

E

embryo 15, 20
emmenagogue 10, 35
emotional disturbances 39
emotions 11, 21, 30
endometriosis 36, 38, 39
endometritis 38
Exeter University 29

F

Fallopian tubes 18, 19, 37, 38
fatigue 36
feelings 21
fibroids 35, 37
flavonoids 25
fluid retention 30, 36, 39
FNIMH 34
follicle-stimulating hormone 16, 17, 18, 19, 27
forgetfulness 36
frequent periods 34
FSH see *follicle-stimulating hormone*

G

Galen 10, 14, 41
Gerard 11, 12
Gerard House 29
Germany 25, 27, 30, 40
GnRH see *gonadotrophin releasing hormone*
gonadotrophin releasing hormone 18, 26, 34, 41
Government monograph 30
Greece, ancient 10
gynaecologist 33

H

headache 36
heavy periods 35, 36
Hera 9
herbalists 33, 34, 43
herbals 10
herpes virus 40
Hippocrates 10, 14, 15, 41
Homer 9
hormone replacement therapy 22, 25, 33, 39, 40
hormones 16, 18, 19, 20, 21, 22, 26, 30, 34, 39
hot flushes 39
HRT see *hormone replacement therapy*
hypothalamus 16, 18, 30, 34, 41

I

implantation 19, 20
infection 22, 38
infertility 26, 27, 28, 36, 37, 38
insomnia 36
insulin 21, 33
iridoids 25
irregular periods 34
irritability 36

L

lactation 18, 21, 31, 39
LH *see luteinising hormone*
libido 14, 19, 21, 41
liver disease 11, 40
Lonicerus 11
lump 33
lunar 14, 15
luteinising hormone 16, 17,
   18, 19, 26, 27, 34, 41

M

males 41
medieval reputation 10
medical herbalists 33, 34, 43
menopausal problems 39
menopause 22
menorrhagia 35
menstrual cycle 14, 16, 18,
   19, 20, 22, 27, 37, 38, 39
menstrual problems 11, 26
milk production 11, 16, 21,
   26
Mittelschmerz 38
MNIMH 34
monk's pepper 10
mood swings 36

N

National Institute of
   Medical Herbalists 34
negative feedback 18
nervous tension 36
North American herbs 14

O

obstetrician 33
obstruction 33

oestrogens 16, 17, 18, 19
öophoritis 38
ovarian cysts 26, 36, 38
ovary 16, 20, 38
ovulation 19, 20, 26, 34, 38
ovum 17, 18, 19
oxytocin 16, 21

P

pain 33, 38
painful periods 35, 36, 38
palpitations 36
pelvic inflammatory disease
   38
pharmacology 25
pheromones 14
Pill, the 33
pinene 25
pituitary 16, 18, 19, 21, 26,
   31, 34, 41
placebo 28, 29, 30
placenta 19, 20, 21
Pliny 9
PMS *see premenstrual
   syndrome*
positive feedback 19, 20
pregnancy 14, 15, 19, 20,
   21, 23, 35, 39
premenstrual syndrome 27,
   29, 30, 35, 36
primary follicle 18
progesterone 16, 17, 19, 21,
   26, 27, 28, 34, 36, 37, 39,
   41
prolactin 16, 21
proof 28
puberty 15, 22, 35

R

Rome, ancient 10

S

sabinene 25
salpingitis 38
science 15, 25, 28
self-examination 33
self-treatment 33, 34
sesquiterpenes 25
shingles 40
side-effects 31
sperm 17, 20, 37
spleen 10, 40
steroidal hormones 16
surgery 37, 38

T

taboo 14
temperature chart 34
testicles 16
testosterone 16, 17, 19, 21,
   22, 41
Thermophona 9
thyroid 16
tincture 43

V

vagina 18
vaginal discharges 34
Vestal virgins 9
vis medicatrix naturae 15
vitamin B1 26
volatile oil 25

W

weight gain 36
wise woman 11
witch-doctor 11
womb 11, 15, 18, 19, 20,
   21, 26, 35, 37, 38
wounds 10, 11, 40

OTHER BOOKS FROM AMBERWOOD PUBLISHING ARE:

Aromatherapy Lexicon – The Essential Reference by Geoff Lyth and Sue Charles is a colourful, fun way to learn about Aromatherapy. £4.99.

Aromatherapy – The Baby Book by Marion Del Gaudio Mak. An easy to follow guide to massage for the infant or child. £3.99

Aromatherapy – Simply For You by Marion Del Gaudio Mak. A clear, simple and comprehensive guide to Aromatherapy for beginners. £1.99.

Aromatherapy – A Guide for Home Use by Christine Westwood. All you need to know about essential oils and using them. £1.99.

Aromatherapy – for Stress Management by Christine Westwood. Covering the use of essential oils for everyday stress-related problems. £3.50.

Aromatherapy – For Healthy Legs and Feet by Christine Westwood. A guide to the use of essential oils for the treatment of legs and feet. £2.99.

Aromatherapy – The Pregnancy Book by Jennie Supper RM RN MGCP. Jennie Supper, a State Registered Nurse and Midwife explains the use of Aromatherapy during pregnancy and the common conditions which may be treated safely. £5.99

Aromatherapy – A Nurses Guide by Ann Percival SRN. The ultimate, safe, lay guide to the natural benefits of Aromatherapy. Including recipes and massage techniques for many medical conditions and a quick reference chart. £2.99.

Aromatherapy – A Nurses Guide for Women by Ann Percival SRN. Concentrates on women's health for all ages. Including sections on PMT, menopause, infertility, cellulite. £2.99.

Aromatherapy – Essential Oils in Colour by Rosemary Caddy Bsc Hons, ARCS MISP is a unique book depicting the chemistry of essential oils. £9.99.

Aroma Science – The Chemistry & Bioactivity of Essential Oils by Dr Maria Lis-Balchin. With a comprehensive list of the Oils and scientific analysis. Includes sections on the sense of smell and the history of Aromatherapy. £4.99.

Plant Medicine – A Guide for Home Use (New Edition) by Charlotte Mitchell MNIMH. A guide to home use giving an insight into the wonderful healing qualities of plants. £2.99.

Ancient Medicine – Ginkgo Biloba (New Edition) by Dr Desmond Corrigan BSc(Pharms), MA, Phd, FLS, FPSI. Improved memory, circulation and concentration are associated with Ginkgo and explained in this book. £2.99.

Indian Medicine – The Immune System by Dr Desmond Corrigan BSc(Pharms), MA, Phd, FLS, FPSI. An intriguing account of the history of the plant called Echinacea and its power to influence the immune system. £2.99.

Herbal Medicine for Sleep & Relaxation by Dr Desmond Corrigan BSc(Pharms), MA, PhD, FLS, FPSI. A guide to the natural sedatives as an alternative to orthodox drug therapies, drawing on the latest medical research, presented in an easy reference format. £2.99.

Herbal First Aid by Andrew Chevallier BA, MNIMH. A beautifully clear reference book of natural remedies and general first aid in the home. £2.99.

Natural Taste – Herbal Teas, A Guide for Home Use by Andrew Chevallier BA, MNIMH. Contains a comprehensive compendium of Herbal Teas gives information on how to make it, its benefits, history and folklore. £3.50.

Garlic– How Garlic Protects Your Heart by Prof E. Ernst MD, PhD. Used as a medicine for over 4500 years, this book examines the latest scientific evidence supporting Garlic's effect in reducing cardiovascular disease, the Western World's number one killer. £3.99.

Phytotherapy – Fifty Vital Herbs by Andrew Chevallier, the most popular medicinal herbs with uses and advice written by an expert. £6.99

Insomnia – Doctor I Can't Sleep by Dr Adrian Williams FRCP. Written by one of the world's leading sleep experts, Dr Williams explains the phenomenon of sleep and sleeping disorders and gives advice on treatment. With 25% of the adult population reporting difficulties sleeping – this book will be essential reading for many. £2.99.

Signs & Symptoms of Vitamin Deficiency by Dr Leonard Mervyn BSc, PhD, C.Chem, FRCS. A home guide for self diagnosis which explains and assesses Vitamin Therapy for the prevention of a wide variety of diseases and illnesses. £2.99.

Causes & Prevention of Vitamin Deficiency by Dr Leonard Mervyn BSc, PhD, C.Chem, FRCS. A home guide to the Vitamin content of foods and the depletion caused by cooking, storage and processing. It includes advice for those whose needs are increased due to lifestyle, illness etc. £2.99.

Eyecare Eyewear – For Better Vision by Mark Rossi Bsc, MBCO. A complete guide to eyecare and eyewear including an assessment of the types of spectacles and contact lenses available and the latest corrective surgical procedures. £3.99.

Arthritis and Rheumatism by Dr John Cosh FRCP, MD. Covers all forms of Arthritis, its effects and the treatments available. £4.95.